Taking to Scale
IMCI Implementation in Mongolia
2000–2008

Lessons Learnt

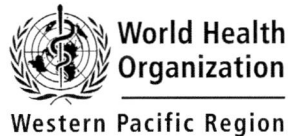

WHO Library Cataloguing in Publication Data

Taking to scale IMCI implementation in Mongolia, 2000-2008 : lessons learnt

1. Child health. 2. Child mortality – prevention and control. 3. Disease management. 4. Mongolia

ISBN 978 92 9061 477 7   (NLM Classification: WA 320)

© **World Health Organization 2011**

All rights reserved. Publications of the World Health Organization can be obtained from WHO Press, World Health Organization, 20 Avenue Appia, 1211 Geneva 27, Switzerland (tel.: +41 22 791 3264; fax: +41 22 791 4857; e-mail: bookorders@who.int). Requests for permission to reproduce or translate WHO publications – whether for sale or for noncommercial distribution – should be addressed to WHO Press, at the above address (fax: +41 22 791 4806; e-mail: permissions@who.int). For WHO Western Pacific Regional Publications, request for permission to reproduce should be addressed to the Publications Office, World Health Organization, Regional Office for the Western Pacific, P.O. Box 2932, 1000, Manila, Philippines, (fax: +632 521 1036, e-mail: publications@wpro.who.int).

The designations employed and the presentation of the material in this publication do not imply the expression of any opinion whatsoever on the part of the World Health Organization concerning the legal status of any country, territory, city or area or of its authorities, or concerning the delimitation of its frontiers or boundaries. Dotted lines on maps represent approximate border lines for which there may not yet be full agreement.

The mention of specific companies or of certain manufacturers' products does not imply that they are endorsed or recommended by the World Health Organization in preference to others of a similar nature that are not mentioned. Errors and omissions excepted, the names of proprietary products are distinguished by initial capital letters.

All reasonable precautions have been taken by the World Health Organization to verify the information contained in this publication. However, the published material is being distributed without warranty of any kind, either expressed or implied. The responsibility for the interpretation and use of the material lies with the reader. In no event shall the World Health Organization be liable for damages arising from its use.

Contents

Foreword	iv
1 Background	1
2 Child health status	2
3 IMCI orientation	7
4 IMCI adaptation	11
5 Planning implementation of IMCI	15
6 Experience with implementation	20
7 Directions for the future	54
Acknowledgement	57

Foreword

The Integrated Management of Childhood Illness (IMCI) strategy was first introduced in the Western Pacific Region in the mid-1990s. It was adopted as a key approach for delivering preventive and treatment interventions that address the most common causes of mortality in newborns, infants and children in 14 countries of the Region. The WHO/UNICEF Regional Child Survival Strategy, endorsed by the WHO Regional Committee during its fifty-sixth session in 2005, focuses on the implementation of a set of seven evidence-based interventions for child survival, including IMCI. It is recognized that the effective implementation of IMCI will contribute to the attainment of Millennium Development Goal 4 to reduce child mortality.

Mongolia was one of the first countries in the Region to implement IMCI and to successfully take it to scale. In particular, the approach used in Mongolia resulted in a common understanding by all stakeholders of the need for IMCI and the implications for systematic and strong support from the health system. Subsequently, IMCI has been successfully incorporated into routine national and subnational planning for child health, making it more likely to be sustainable in the longer term. This document reviews the process of IMCI implementation in Mongolia. It is hoped that the experiences and lessons learnt are relevant to all countries introducing IMCI or planning further expansion.

Shin Young-soo, MD, Ph.D.
Regional Director

1 Background

Mongolia has made good progress in reducing infant and child mortality since 1990. The National Programme for the Development and Protection of Children 2002–2010 outlines the Government's approach to achieving the Millennium Development Goal (MDG) 4 child-mortality targets set in the United Nations General Assembly Special Session in 2002. Improving the health status of mothers and children is also given priority in the Health Sector Strategic Master Plan 2006–2015 and the medium-term expenditure framework. Recent mortality data show that Mongolia is on track to achieve its MDG for child health.

The Integrated Management of Childhood Illness (IMCI) approach was begun in Mongolia in 2000. By the end of 2006, IMCI implementation had been extended to all provinces in the country. IMCI was subsequently included as a key approach in the national strategic plan for child health.

A review of the child health programme in 2007 found that a number of lessons had been learnt in the early implementation phase of IMCI that have resulted in more effective programming. This report summarizes the lessons learnt and directions for the future.

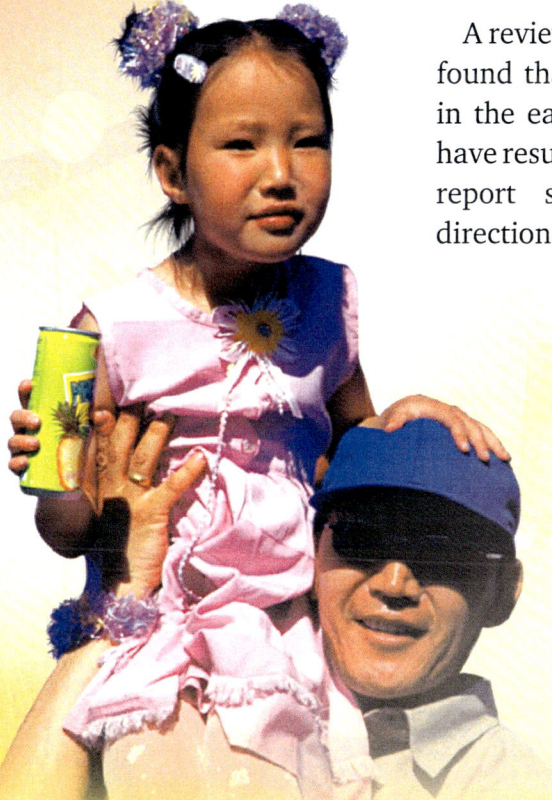

2 Child Health Status

The epidemiological profile of child deaths in Mongolia, and the relatively high prevalence of stunting and micronutrient deficiencies, resulted in IMCI being selected as a key approach for preventing and managing childhood illness. Data on child health status were important in adapting IMCI to the local context and planning for IMCI implementation.

2.1 Morbidity and mortality

Overall, child mortality has shown a downward trend since 1990[1] (see Figure 1), with most of the mortality decline in children aged 12 to 59 months. However, the proportion of all under-five deaths that take place in the neonatal period has risen over time and is estimated to be 36%[2]. Mortality rates show substantial variations between subpopulations, with rates higher in the western areas of the country, in rural areas, and among the migratory population. The most important causes of child mortality in 2006 were perinatal

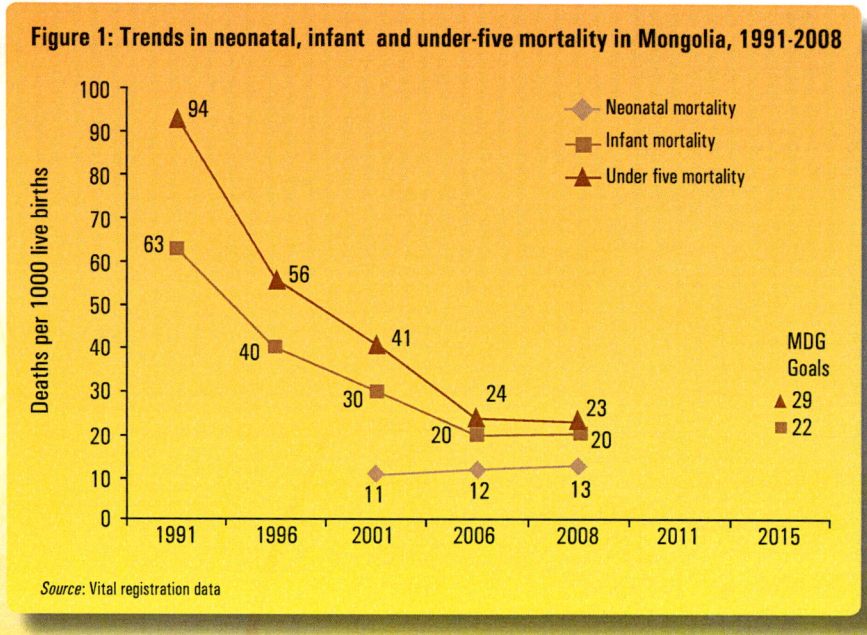

Figure 1: Trends in neonatal, infant and under-five mortality in Mongolia, 1991-2008

Source: Vital registration data

[1] Mongolia vital reporting data, 2007
[2] *Global burden of disease: 2004 update*. Geneva, World Health Organization, 2008

causes (37%), acute respiratory tract infections (ARI) (20%), injuries (13%) and diarrhoea (5%)[3] (see Figure 2). The main causes of neonatal mortality were asphyxia (39%), prematurity (31%), congenital problems (15%) and infections (13%). The prevalence of low birth weight was estimated to be 8% in 1998 and 5% in 2008[4].

ARI was estimated to be responsible for more than half of child deaths in 1996 and for 38% in 1998, just before IMCI was initiated. At that time, ARI was estimated to be the reason for 25%–39% of visits to health facilities and for 33% of hospital admissions. In 1998, about 9%–10% of deaths were reported to be caused by diarrhoeal diseases; diarrhoeal morbidity was thought to be underreported, because many cases were treated at home. The proportion of child deaths caused by diarrhoea has decreased over time, while the proportion caused by injuries has increased.

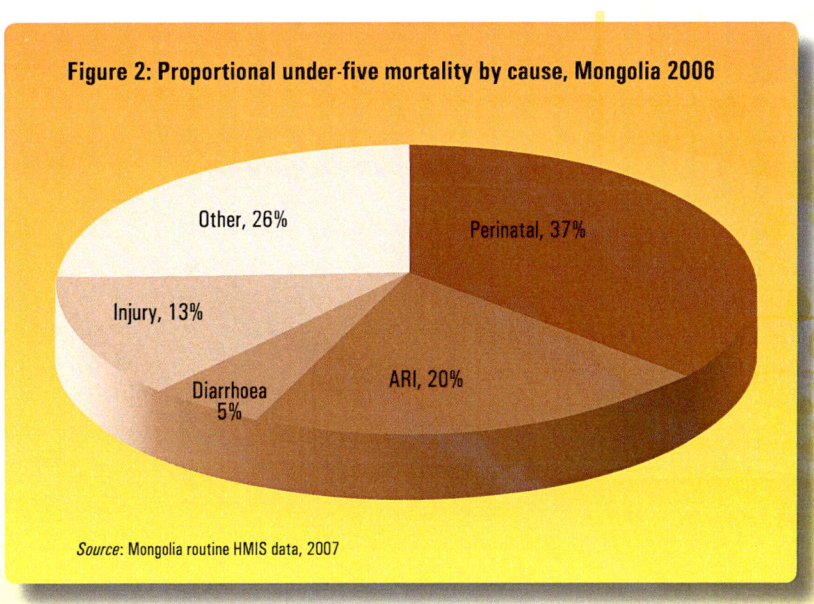

Figure 2: Proportional under-five mortality by cause, Mongolia 2006

Other, 26%
Perinatal, 37%
Injury, 13%
Diarrhoea 5%
ARI, 20%

Source: Mongolia routine HMIS data, 2007

[3]Mongolia routine Health Management Information System (HMIS) data, 2007
[4]United Nations Population Fund (UNFPA) Reproductive Health Survey (RHS), 2008

2.2 Nutrition

In general, rates of wasting, underweight and stunting fell between 1992 and 2005 (see Figure 3). In 2005, 21% of children were estimated to be stunted (below -2SD of normal height for age), 2% were wasted (below -2SD of normal weight for height) and 6% were underweight (below -2SD weight for age)[5]. Rural populations have higher rates than urban populations on all nutrition markers. Rates of stunting have fallen less rapidly than those for wasting and underweight, and remain relatively high. Stunting is an indicator of chronic undernutrition and suggests that long-term nutrient intake is inadequate. Stunting is most prevalent in the 6-24 months age group, suggesting that weaning practices need to be improved.

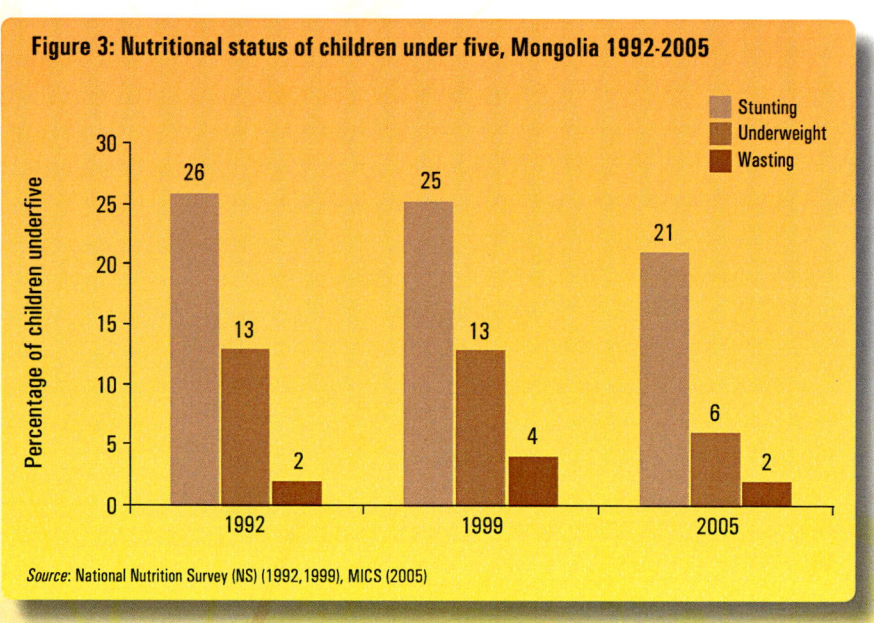

Figure 3: Nutritional status of children under five, Mongolia 1992-2005

Source: National Nutrition Survey (NS) (1992,1999), MICS (2005)

[5] Multiple Indicator Cluster Survey (MICS), 2005

The proportion of children who are anaemic declined by almost half between 1999 and 2004, although 22% of children were still found to be anaemic in 2004. Despite a diet apparently high in protein and bioavailable iron, anaemia is a major problem. The prevalence of anaemia varies significantly in different age groups, begins early in infancy and peaks at 12-18 months. The most common cause of anaemia is considered to be iron deficiency, but lack of dietary folate is also thought to contribute.

The proportion of children with goitre declined from 21% to 14% between 2000 and 2004, suggesting that the consumption of iodized salt improved.

Rickets is a major child health problem. A survey in 1997 found that at least one of the three signs of rickets (rachitic rosary, Harrison´s groove or enlarged size of fontanel) was present in 68% of children under five years of age[6]. The high prevalence of rickets is believed to be due to the limited exposure to ultraviolet light during the winter months, cold weather for most of the year limiting skin exposure, the cultural emphasis on infant swaddling and the limited availability of foods rich in vitamin D. Seasonally, low calcium intake and factors inhibiting calcium absorption also may contribute to the high prevalence of rickets.

A programme for prevention and treatment, "Stoss therapie", began in 1993. The programme strategy was to distribute vitamin D supplements (50 000 IU) to children from birth to two years of age. However, the 1997 rickets survey found that only 33% of children had received a dose of vitamin D in the previous six months. No change was seen in the proportion of children with a low serum vitamin D between 1999 and 2004, with the rate remaining around 40% overall and higher in western regions of the country.

[6] Nutrition Research Center/World Vision International Rickets Survey, 1997

The proportion of children aged 6-59 months who had received a vitamin A dose within the last six months doubled from 32% in 2000 to 65% in 2005. Supplementation is highest in Ulaanbaatar and lowest in the western region of the country.[7] A serosurvey in 2006 found that 33% of children aged 6-36 months had serum retinol below the norm. Since the usual Mongolian diet is often deficient in foods containing vitamin A, it is assumed that subclinical vitamin A deficiency is likely to be a problem. The proportion of mothers who received a high dose vitamin A supplement within eight weeks of giving birth quadrupled from 13% in 2000 to 56% in 2005. Supplementation of mothers is highest in Ulaanbaatar and lowest in the western region.

Lessons learnt: Introducing IMCI
Use local child health data to make planning decisions

- Malaria was not a significant cause of morbidity and mortality and was removed from the Mongolian adaptation of the generic IMCI guidelines.
- Newborn deaths were an important component of all child deaths; prevention and management of newborn illness needed to be a programme focus.
- Rates of stunting and micronutrient deficiencies (iron, iodine, vitamin D, vitamin A) remained high. Improving the feeding practices of caretakers in the home needed to be emphasized and guidelines on the management of vitamin D deficiency were needed.
- There were a number of high-risk groups such as western areas of the country, rural areas, migrant populations that needed to be reached.

[7] MICS, 2005

IMCI Orientation

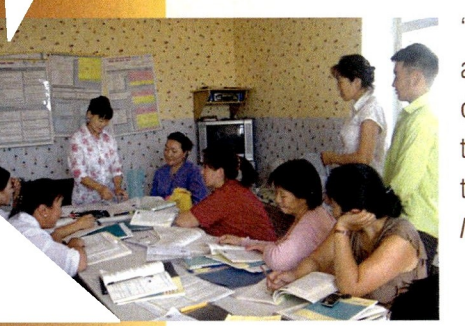

"Because we had all those involved with child health around the table from the beginning, we made decisions together. Nothing was a surprise. We knew that we had the full support of staff at the top and at the bottom. That was important for making IMCI work."
IMCI focal person, Ulaanbaatar

The IMCI orientation meeting was held in Ulaanbaatar City from 24 to 25 June 1999. Its objective was to reach a common understanding on the concepts and principles of the IMCI strategy and its implications for the health care system. During the meeting, options for organizing and coordinating IMCI implementation were discussed, including possible resource requirements. Approaches to improving collaboration between child health-related programmes and departments in the Ministry of Health were reviewed, as well as the implications of IMCI for the Health Sector Development Programme supported by the Asian Development Bank (ADB). The meeting was organized by the Ministry of Health in collaboration with WHO and the United Nations Children's Fund (UNICEF).

The orientation meeting brought together child health-related staff in the Ministry of Health from the national and *aimag* levels, as well as representatives from training institutions, professional groups, multilateral and bilateral partners, and nongovernmental organizations (NGOs). It provided an opportunity to share information and experience as regards the content and implications of the IMCI strategy with a wide range of stakeholders, and to get their input.

By the end of the orientation meeting, agreement had been reached in several areas:

- **The importance of improving health workers' skills, health systems and family and community practices in a balanced way** in order to ensure the effectiveness and sustainability of child health activities.

- **The need to link the introduction of IMCI to health sector reform activities**. A programme on health sector development, supported by ADB, was initiated in 1998 with the objective of re-orienting the health care delivery system to an approach more oriented towards primary health care. The strategies used included strengthened family group units, training and curriculum development for family doctors and nurses in women's and children's health, and introduction of a funding scheme, including a component for supplies and equipment. It was agreed that the IMCI strategy could be closely linked to those reforms by providing the technical basis for high quality and cost-effective health services.

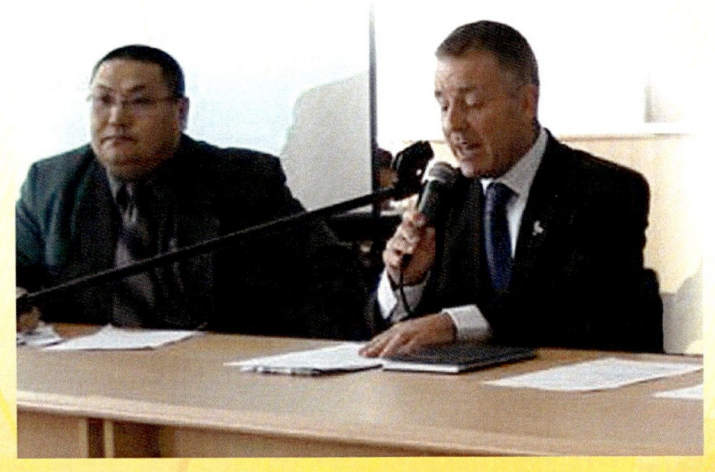

- **The need for a coordinating group within the Ministry of Health**. It was agreed that a high-level steering committee would be formed to oversee implementation, while a technical working group would be responsible for implementation, with an IMCI focal person in charge of the working group. Prior to 1991, child health activities were included in the Control of Diarrhoeal Diseases (CDD) and ARI programmes, established in Mongolia in 1983 and 1991, respectively. Those programmes were combined in 1991. The introduction of IMCI needed to link with these existing programmes.

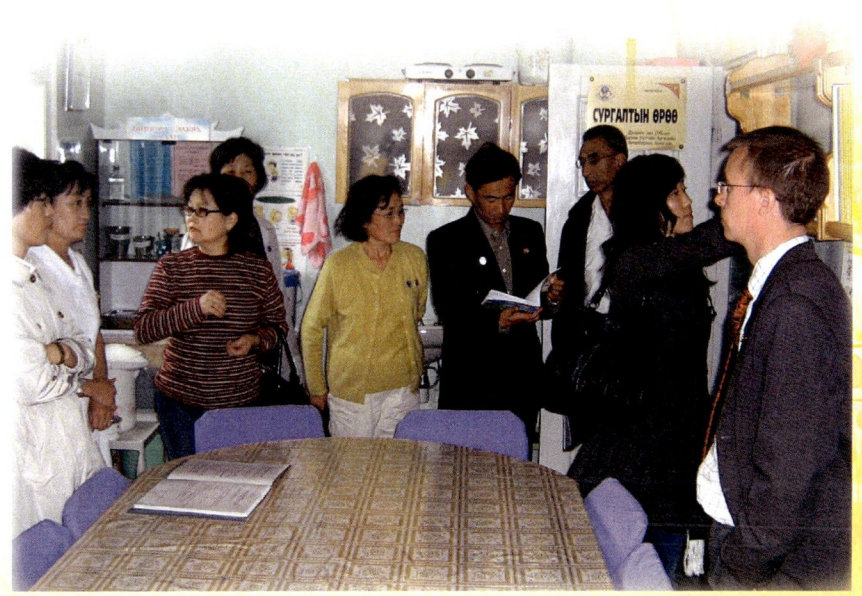

- **The need for continued involvement of all stakeholders, including staff from within the Ministry of Health, as well as donors and other partners, in order for implementation to succeed**. At the orientation meeting, all stakeholders expressed their commitment to incorporating IMCI into their own child health plans, and WHO and UNICEF committed to providing technical support and funds for early implementation. A Mongolian name for IMCI was discussed and agreed upon.

- **The next steps, including development of an implementation plan and adaptation of the IMCI guidelines**. It was agreed that working groups were needed to adapt the IMCI guidelines for the local context.

Lessons learnt: IMCI orientation

Ensure IMCI orientation is conducted early to:

- inform Ministry of Health staff about the IMCI approach and why it could be an effective intervention for reducing child mortality;
- obtain the commitment and support of stakeholders who could provide financial, human and material resources to support implementation;
- reach agreement on the organizational structure needed to implement IMCI, including a steering committee, a working group and a focal person; and
- make a decision on next steps, including how to plan implementation and adapt the IMCI guidelines for the local context.

4 IMCI Adaptation

> "When we began IMCI some people were skeptical, particularly doctors. They were not sure whether it was right for Mongolia. Then we got them involved with the adaptation and they saw that they could make changes and they could debate how it should work. Then they were more comfortable. That made a big difference to how they saw it. Then they gave their support."
> *Paediatrician*, Ulaanbaatar

A workshop to begin the process of IMCI adaptation and to plan early implementation was conducted from 10 to 13 August 1999. At that workshop, the IMCI steering committee, working group and focal person were announced. The ARI/CDD programme manager became the IMCI focal person. Workshop participants were divided into two groups: one to develop an implementation plan and one to review adaptations to the generic IMCI guidelines. Participants included members of the IMCI steering committee and working group, *aimag* staff and donors. A consensus-building meeting was held later to reach agreement on the draft plan and the draft adaptations.

Adaptation of IMCI clinical guidelines

The adaptation group reviewed the IMCI clinical guidelines. After major issues had been identified, two subgroups were formed: the "Diseases group" to address ARI, diarrhoea, fever, ear problems and rickets; and the "Nutrition and young infant group" to address nutrition and the young infant. Tasks were identified and a time schedule to complete them was defined.

Main adaptation tasks included:

- removing conditions from the generic guidelines that were not important public health problems in Mongolia, including measles, HIV/AIDS, hookworm and whipworm infections, borreliosis and malaria (the 'fever' box was adapted for the local context);

- developing guidelines for the assessment, classification, management and follow-up of rickets (development of those guidelines required field-testing);

- reviewing the weight-for-age threshold for classification of children as very low weight-for-age (the -3SD values of the national weight-for-age standard corresponded to -2SD of the National Centre for Health Statistics (NCHS)/WHO standard). Iron and folate were recommended for treatment and prevention of anaemia in children. An iron/folate formulation needed to be added to the essential drug list;

- testing the feasibility and acceptability of local feeding recommendations using a household feeding trial (the tests were conducted by the Nutrition Research Centre);

- reviewing the importance of vitamin A deficiency in children under five, and deciding on the treatment protocols for vitamin A in the management of malnutrition; and

- testing local terms for use in the guidelines and adapting the mother's card.

Rickets – a unique adaptation for Mongolia

Rickets has been identified as a serious public health problem in Mongolia. Although rickets itself is not a fatal disease, it may lead to permanent bone deformity and is associated with impaired growth and development and a reduction in the immune response to infection. Infections like pneumonia (the main cause of death in Mongolian children under five years of age), tuberculosis and diarrhoea are more likely to cause death in rachitic children. The adaptation group felt strongly that the treatment and prevention of rickets should be included in the IMCI guidelines.

Data on the sensitivity, specificity and positive predictive value of clinical rickets signs were not available in Mongolia. Clinical guidelines for prevention and treatment were therefore developed based on the experience of Mongolian clinicians, literature review and discussions with resource persons.

IMCI clinical guidelines for rickets

All children under two years of age are examined for the presence of craniotabes, rib beading, hypotonus and excessive perspiration. The presence of at least one of the signs craniotabes or rib beading and at least one of the signs hypotonus or excessive perspiration indicates "RICKETS" (yellow row) requiring treatment. The absence of these signs indicates "NO RICKETS" (green row) and requires preventive measures. Recommended treatment for rickets is the daily administration of three drops of vitamin D spirit solution (12 000 IU daily, 360 000 IU per month) for 30 days and advice to mothers to expose the child to sunlight, if possible.

The prevention method for rickets is the daily administration of vitamin D water solution (500 IU/drop), starting from the age of one month in term newborns and 14 days in pre-term newborns until the age of two years. An alternative for children aged two months to two years is monthly administration (except for the three summer months) of 50 000 IU vitamin D capsules. Sun exposure is also recommended. Dietary measures aimed at the improvement of vitamin D and calcium intake are included in feeding recommendations.

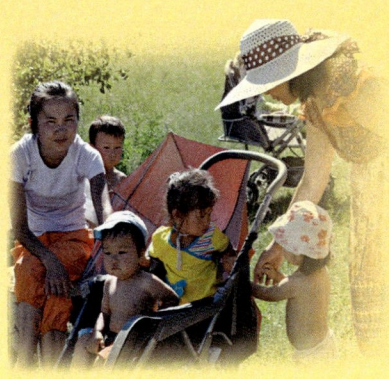
IMCI guidelines support preventive measures by ensuring that vitamin D is taken, recommending sun exposure and giving feeding recommendations. *Feldshers* play a key role in prevention. They conduct monthly visits to children less than one year of age and several visits to children between one and two years of age.

The community component of IMCI also supports rickets prevention by organizing "summer camps" with the cooperation of the local health authorities. This means gathering of all children under two (with their mothers) in a given community every day during the summer months. Sunbathing is organized at these gatherings and children who are not exclusively breastfed receive milk and milk products. These gatherings also serve as breastfeeding peer support groups and allow health education.

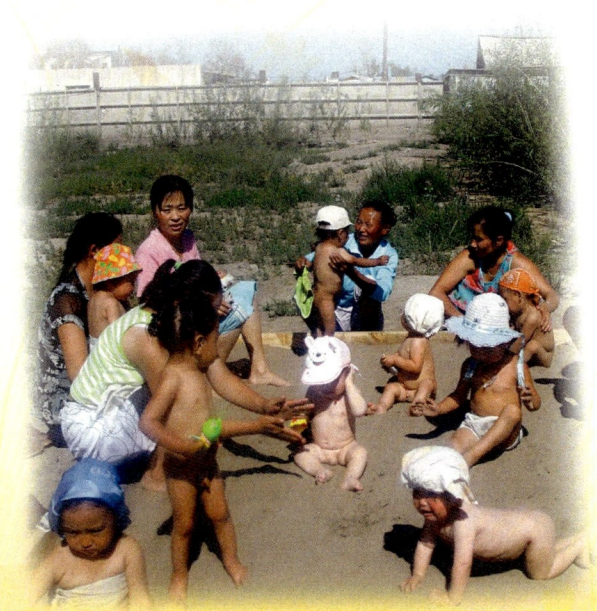

5. Planning Implementation of IMCI

By the end of 2006, IMCI had been implemented in all provinces in the country (see Figure 4). There were two key elements to effective implementation planning in Mongolia: the development of a national IMCI implementation plan for the early implementation phase that was fully funded; and a process of annual review and planning, done in collaboration with *aimag* staff.

5.1 Development of a national IMCI implementation plan

This was done by an implementation planning group, comprising members of the IMCI working group and donors. The plan included the following elements:

- **Selection of focus areas for early implementation.** Arhangai *aimag*, Ovorhangai *aimag* (UNICEF-supported),

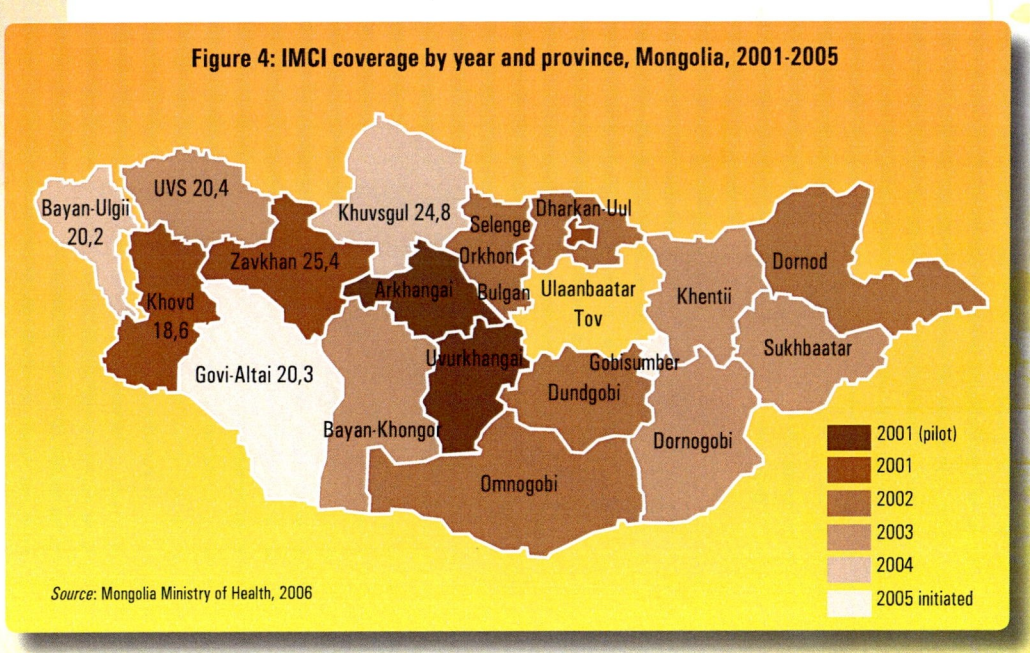

Figure 4: IMCI coverage by year and province, Mongolia, 2001-2005

Source: Mongolia Ministry of Health, 2006

Songinokhairhan district (World Vision-supported), and Sukhbaatar district (ADB-supported) were selected for the early implementation phase. Lessons learnt in these areas were used to plan further training in other areas.

- **Selection of target groups for in-service training**. *Bagh feldshers*, family doctors in *aimags* and district health centres and *soum* hospital doctors were selected as the target groups for training. *Bagh feldshers* provide primary health care services to villages and households, family doctors provide outpatient care at first-level facilities and *soum* doctors provide referral level care in *soums*. Since family nurses work closely with family doctors, it was agreed that the IMCI implementation group should also train them in IMCI so that they could support family doctors.

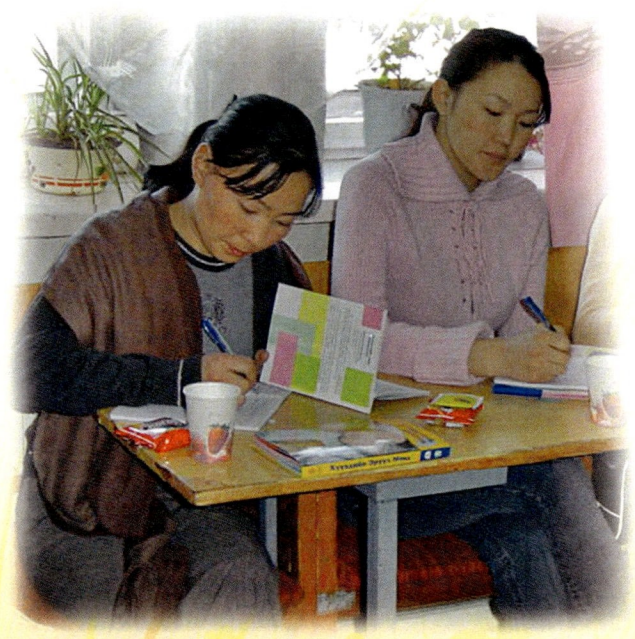

- **An in-service training plan**. The training plan was important to ensure that an adequate number of facilitators and health workers were trained, and that the quality of the training was adequate.
- **A review of the essential drug list and drug availability in the implementation areas**. It was agreed that essential IMCI drugs must be made available in implementation areas.
- **An approach to supervision**. It was agreed that the existing supervisory system would be used. Supervisors would use methods developed for follow-up after IMCI training. At *soum* level, it was recommended that all *bagh feldshers* should visit *soum* hospitals once a month to report on their activities. The IMCI implementation group planned to discuss further how to use these visits to reinforce the skills of health workers.
- **An estimated budget for early implementation activities**. Budget lines were allocated to donors: WHO, UNICEF, ADB and World Vision International. This ensured that resources were available for all activities in advance, and allowed effective planning.

Lessons learnt: Planning

Establish criteria for selection of early implementation areas

- Good physical access to central-level staff
- Committed staff in the *aimags* and districts to do planning and management
- Availability of a suitable training site
- Availability of drugs needed for implementation of IMCI in health facilities
- Referral-level care available
- Availability of other resources to support the IMCI strategy

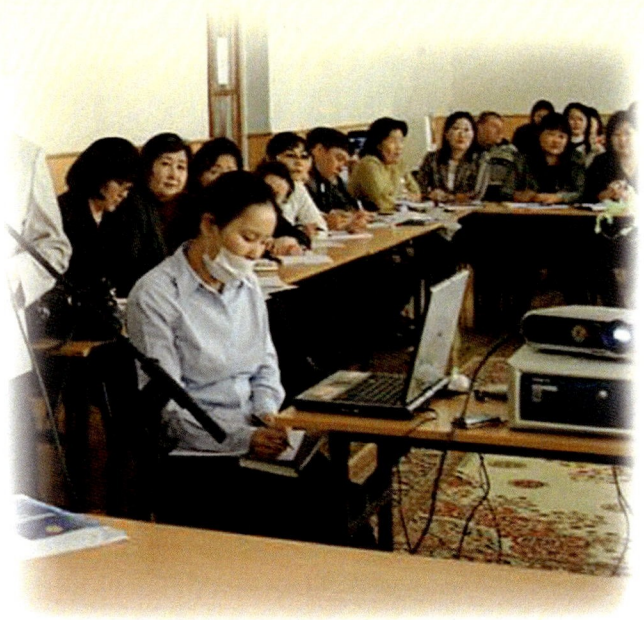

5.2 Annual review and planning with *aimag* staff

The process to review the performance of the previous year and plan activities for the coming year began in 2001. *Aimag* managers and national staff meet together to review routine data and activities conducted in their own areas. This allows local managers to highlight problems or gaps and make decisions how to overcome them, and gives national managers a clear idea of how implementation is progressing at the lower levels. Routine data reviewed include mortality, morbidity, immunization coverage and training coverage. Managers can compare data from each *soum* in their own areas. This process has proved to be very useful for addressing gaps and problems, and for trying to match available resources with those areas where they are most needed. The responsibilities of each level are clearly defined, with the national level responsible for planning and orientation meetings, pre-service training, and translation, adaptation and printing of training materials. The *aimag* level uses local budgets to support local in-service health worker training and follow-up, supervision and provision of equipment and supplies.

Over time, it has become clear that *aimag* managers often do not have experience in using data for programme decision-making, and their skills in this area need to be improved. In addition, data on how well child health-related activities have been implemented (programme outputs) are not always collected at the lower level. Improvements in this area would provide even more information for planning. Early training for local managers in planning skills would have helped facilitate IMCI implementation even further.

Lessons learnt: Planning

Plan IMCI with stakeholders

- A fully funded national implementation plan, developed with stakeholders, was critical for the early implementation phase.
- Phased implementation, beginning in a few areas, allowed lessons to be learnt that were useful for further expansion.
- Annual planning with *aimag* staff allowed planning to be done more effectively. Problems and funding needs could be identified, and workplans for the next year were developed collaboratively.
- The planning skills of *aimag* staff are important for implementation of IMCI. Improved planning skills would allow them to implement activities more effectively.

Experience with Implementation

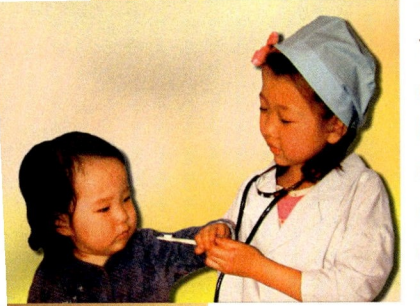

"IMCI was put into the four-year government plan of action. This meant that it was endorsed by the Government, and everyone could see that. Then there were decrees issued for expanding IMCI in the country. That was quite important, because then everyone, including the health workers could see that it was part of their job. Health workers have to think of it as part of their job, otherwise they will not take it so seriously."
Soum family doctor

6.1 Policies and guidelines

Several areas of policy were important in supporting or facilitating IMCI implementation. Many are general policy areas crucial for all child health-related activities. The policy areas supporting IMCI implementation included:

- **General policies and laws**. The National Programme for the Development and Protection of Children 2002–2010 and the Health Sector Strategic Master Plan 2006–2015 both include IMCI as a key strategy and require a proportion of the child health budget to be allocated to IMCI activities. In addition, decrees were issued to support the adoption and expansion of IMCI. Several other laws have proved relevant in improving child health, including those on hygiene and sanitation standards, the iodization of salt, and the required immunization schedule for children. Mongolia ratified the Convention on the Rights of the Child in 1990, and fulfills its reporting requirements.

- **Programme strategies**. Several other programmes had strategies that were important for reducing child morbidity and mortality and were closely linked with IMCI, including: the Maternal Mortality Reduction Strategy; the National Strategy for Prevention of Micronutrient Deficiency among Mothers and Children; the National Infant and Young Child Feeding (IYCF) Strategy; and the Growth Monitoring Promotion Strategy for children under three years old.

- **The International Code for Marketing Breast-milk Substitutes**. The code has been adopted by Mongolia, although it is recognized that further work is needed to properly enforce it. Monitoring how well the code is applied by producers and distributors of breast-milk substitutes involves regular review of the product labelling and advertising used by formula manufacturers. A functioning monitoring system should include: (1) enough staff to conduct regular monitoring; (2) clear channels for reporting violations; and (3) clear actions to be taken when violations are detected.

- **Technical guidelines**. IMCI technical guidelines were updated as new information became available. Important technical updates included: the inclusion of zinc and low osmolarity oral rehydration salts (ORS) for the management of diarrhoea; the addition of the management of the sick newborn from birth; and the modification of the period for exclusive breastfeeding from four months to six months (the duration of exclusive breastfeeding was changed in 2002).

- **Revision of the essential drug list** to ensure that it included IMCI medications, including pre-referral drugs.

- **Policies to ensure the financial protection of infants and children**. Since 2000, there has been a steady increase in the state budget for the health sector, both in terms of percentage of gross domestic product (GDP) and of government expenditure. The main financing sources in 2005 were the state budget (69%), the health insurance fund (23%) and out-of-pocket payments and other sources (4%). Total health expenditure was 4% of GDP in 2005.

Health care financing resources are spent on hospital-based curative services and preventive health services. In 2005, 28% of total health expenditures were spent on tertiary health care facilities, 43% on secondary health care facilities, such as *aimag* and district general hospitals, and 29% on primary health care facilities. A greater allocation for primary health care is needed.

Currently, caretakers are required to pay for drugs at first-level facilities. Since medications at referral hospitals are still provided free of charge, the result has been an increase in the number of patients going straight to this level for basic services. The policy discourages the use of primary clinics and needs to be re-examined. Infants and children should have access to care, regardless of the ability of their caretakers to pay.

All health services for children under 18 years of age are free of charge. The health insurance system was introduced in 1994 and, by 2005, covered 73% of the population. Primary health care services were initially paid by the health insurance fund. However, since a significant proportion of caretakers could not afford insurance coverage, particularly poor and vulnerable groups, access to primary health care was limited by that approach. In July 2006, the Health Law was changed to ensure that all primary health care services are financed from the state budget, and are not dependent on insurance membership. Access to primary health care is still limited for some migrant groups, however, because they need to be registered with the local government in order to receive services, which is difficult if they are highly mobile. Strategies for reaching such groups need to be improved.

Lessons learnt: Policies and guidelines

Ensure policies and guidelines support IMCI implementation

- A number of general policies and laws are important in supporting the implementation of IMCI. These include the health sector strategy and decrees supporting IMCI expansion.
- Other programmes help to disseminate IMCI technical standards. These include nutrition, maternal and newborn programmes.
- Technical guidelines for IMCI, including the essential drug list, need to be reviewed regularly and updated if necessary.
- Monitoring of how well the International Code of Marketing Breast-milk Substitutes is applied by producers and distributors needs to be improved.
- While attempts have been made to improve the financing of primary health care services from the state budget for poor and migrating populations, these populations cannot access services in some areas. Implementation of financing policies needs to be reviewed regularly.

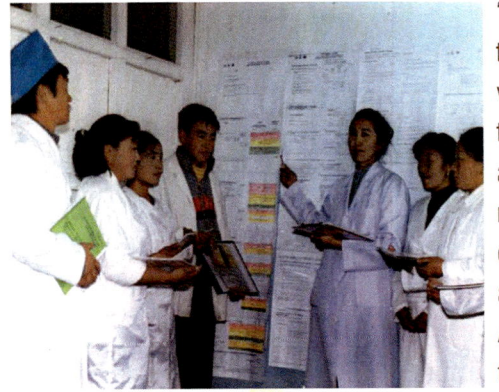

"We have quite successfully expanded IMCI in-service training because we made a training plan early on. This plan was funded from the outset. This meant that we could do the training in a systematic way, by training facilitators first, and by being careful to ensure that the quality of training was maintained. Then, as we expanded IMCI, we revised the plan every year. When we had a plan, we could go to the donors and be very specific. This is what is needed, we could say. And because donors could see we had thought it through, they gave funding." *IMCI focal person*, Ulaanbaatar

6.2 Improving the availability of IMCI-trained health workers

In-service training

By 2006, all provinces in the country had implemented IMCI, and 75% of all health workers had received IMCI training. The primary focus of in-service training was *bagh feldshers*, family doctors and *soum* doctors, and the standard 11-day course was used. The in-service training plan, developed as a part of implementation planning, specified: training sites and how they were selected; the standards required for high quality training; how facilitators would be selected; the sequence in which training would be conducted (facilitator training preceded health worker training); and how follow-up visits after training would be carried out. The plan was revised every year as IMCI implementation was expanded. Local terms and feeding recommendations in the adapted IMCI materials were well understood, and feedback from health workers on the quality of training was positive. Three issues emerged in the area of IMCI staff training:

- **Lack of staff in remote and rural areas**. A national human resources policy is available for the period 2004–2013, but it has not yet been able to address the problem of inadequate staff numbers in remote and rural areas. In 2006, 15 *soums* had no doctor available and 90 *baghs* had no *feldsher*. Both of these types of health worker are important to providing effective IMCI. *Feldshers* are particularly important since they are the front-line staff, responsible for home visits and primary health care. The problem of staff distribution is believed to be caused by two factors: (1) there are no incentives to encourage staff to remain in more remote areas; and (2) too many doctors but not enough primary care health workers are being trained. The continued overproduction of doctors has resulted in a high physician-nurse ratio of 1:1.18, and a shortage of nurses, midwives and primary health care personnel. The situation is further compounded by the overspecialization of doctors, which contributes to their shortage at the primary health care level. Once staff have been trained, better methods for retaining them in rural or remote areas are needed. These could include a written

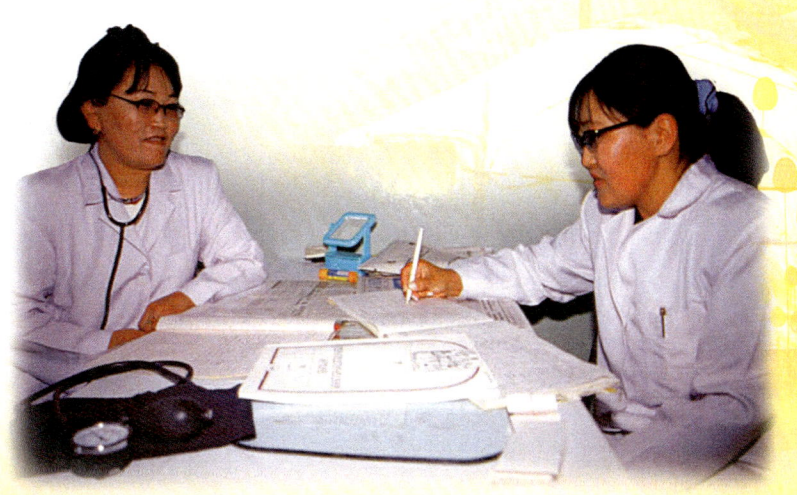

requirement for all newly trained staff to spend a specified period of time in more remote areas, as well as incentives. Incentives could be financial, or could include improved opportunities for training and promotion.

- **Cost of in-service training**. The standard 11-day IMCI training course used in Mongolia has proved to be relatively expensive due to high residential costs. It has been particularly difficult to train all *bagh feldshers* because of their high numbers. There are 971 rural *baghs* in Mongolia, each of which should be serviced by a *feldsher*. Most of the costs of training have been covered by donors. For this reason, a shift towards pre-service training has become a high priority.

- **Difficult to complete follow-up visits after IMCI training**. Follow-up after training has not been done regularly, primarily due to a lack of resources at the lower levels, including trained staff to carry out visits and funding for vehicles, fuel and per diem payments. Local budgets need to allocate more resources for follow-up visits after IMCI training, but it has been difficult to get funds allocated. Local decision-makers need to have greater awareness of the importance of this issue.

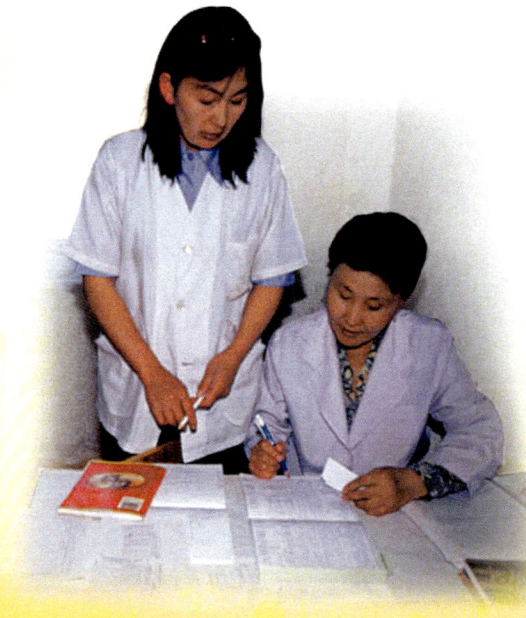

Pre-service training

Pre-service IMCI education was introduced in 2002. A pre-service training team was formed to oversee implementation. IMCI modules were added to the curricula at the Health Science University and at four regional medical colleges. Funding of the introduction of pre-service IMCI training was provided by WHO and the Arabian Gulf Fund (AGFUND), as well as the Ministry of Health. The IMCI handbook and training materials were produced, and IMCI training rooms were equipped and furnished. All training sites now have designated IMCI training centres. Early in the process, a pre-service training course was conducted for lecturers in the key institutions. IMCI is being taught in different ways at different training institutions, as summarized in the box below. A review of pre-service training implementation in November 2005 found that the regular involvement of staff from the academic institutions and professional societies in the introduction and implementation of IMCI was key to getting teaching institutions to adopt it so quickly. Staff from teaching institutions participated in the national IMCI Task Force and IMCI review committees, courses for IMCI master trainers and facilitators, and follow-up visits after

---

Integrating IMCI into pre-service education

- Department of Pediatrics, Health Science University: IMCI is taught in the third, fourth and fifth years and is included in the final examination.

- Department of Family Medicine, Health Science University: IMCI is taught in the sixth year for one week (24 hours).

- Nursing colleges at Ulaanbaatar and Darkhan: IMCI is taught in the second, third and fourth years and is included in the final examination.

- *Feldsher* training at Dornogovi and Govi-altai: IMCI is taught in the second, third and fourth years and is included in the final examination.

IMCI training. This close involvement meant that they understood IMCI, had field experience with it, and believed it useful for training of health staff. It is hoped that, in the long term, there will no longer be a need for in-service training for most health workers.

Issues raised after early experiences with pre-service IMCI training included:

- Large classes sometimes make it difficult for tutors to ensure that all students receive adequate clinical training. This is an ongoing challenge.

- "Block" teaching of IMCI, in which the technical basis of IMCI and clinical training are all given together, is hard to sustain. Many now favour a staggered approach, in which smaller pieces are taught over time, with a five-day synthesis block at the end.

- The quality of pre-service training is not yet being routinely monitored. Methods and indicators for tracking the quality of training are needed.

> **Lessons learnt: Human resources**
>
> **Improve the availability and quality of IMCI-trained health workers**
>
> - Both in-service and pre-service training plans are essential to improving coverage with IMCI-trained health workers. These need to be reviewed and revised regularly.
>
> - The unavailability of trained staff in remote and rural areas is a problem in Mongolia. Child health staff should advocate for training of more primary health staff and for incentives to encourage them to stay where they are needed.
>
> - Follow-up after training will not happen routinely unless it is seen as a part of training and included in local health budgets.
>
> - The involvement of staff from pre-service training institutions in the planning and implementation of IMCI made it quicker and easier to introduce IMCI into the pre-service training curricula of health workers.
>
> - The quality of both pre- and in-service training should be monitored routinely. Methods and indicators for reviewing quality are needed.

6.3 Strengthening health systems

Access to health services

In order for IMCI to be as effective as possible, the caretakers of young children must have access to preventive and treatment services from IMCI-trained providers. Available data from Mongolia suggest that access to many essential health services is high. Approximately 99% of women were estimated to have received at least four antenatal care visits in 2008[8], while the proportion of births assisted by health personnel was 99%.[9] The proportion of children with fast or difficult breathing who were taken to a health facility in 2005 was 63%.[10] The proportion of children under five years who are fully immunized has been consistently high, and was estimated to be 98% in 2006 from routine data. However, access remains limited for some subpopulations, including poor, rural and migratory groups. The main remaining barriers to access are:

- **Geographic**. Approximately 67% of the population of *soums* are nomadic herders; 35% of the nomadic population live 50-80 km from a health facility, while 65% live less than 14 km from a health facility. *Bagh feldshers* are often long distances from the more remote nomadic populations, and it is difficult for them to conduct home visits to all of them regularly.

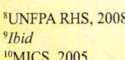

[8]UNFPA RHS, 2008
[9]*Ibid*
[10]MICS, 2005

- **Drug financing policy**. Although services are free of charge for all children under 18 years of age, caretakers have to pay for drugs at first-level facilities. This may discourage care-seeking at the primary care level, particularly for poor households. Since drugs are provided free of charge at referral hospitals, a by-pass effect has been noted, with more caretakers going directly to higher levels. This has increased patient numbers at the referral level and has put pressure on the system.

- **Unavailability of human resources**. Staff are not available in some remote and rural areas. As mentioned in the training section, in 2006, 15 *soums* had no doctor and 90 *baghs* had no *feldsher*. Inadequate numbers of nurses, midwives and primary health doctors are produced. In addition, trained health workers often move away from rural areas to jobs in more urban areas. All these conditions contribute to the lack of health staff at the primary health care level.

- **Health system administration**. Caretakers and children must be registered with the local government system in order to be eligible for services in that area. However, migratory groups are often not registered with local governments in areas where they live for short periods of time, and therefore find it more difficult to get services. This discourages care-seeking and is a barrier to access to health services.

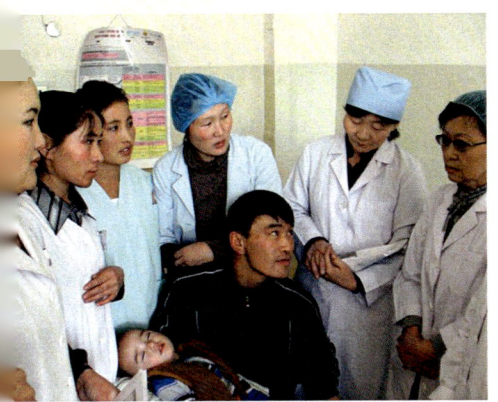

"The health facility survey provided a structured way of looking at what health workers were doing. Before the survey, everyone thought that practice would be perfect because most health workers had been trained in IMCI. Then the survey found that practice was not always so good. It was useful to find this out because it pointed us in the right direction. We could see what needed to be improved, and could work to address the problem. Before the survey, we had no information to work with."
Aimag IMCI facilitator

Quality care

An IMCI health facility survey was conducted in 2006 to review the quality of care at outpatient health facilities. A total of 41 health facilities were sampled from a list of 294 that had implemented IMCI. The results are summarized in Figures 5 and 6. Of the facilities visited, 76% had trained at least 60% of the staff seeing sick children in IMCI. Only 40% of the sick children seen had been weighed and plotted on a growth chart, an essential element of IMCI assessment, while only 34% had been assessed for rickets, a key adaptation added in Mongolia. The low coverage rates of both of these measures suggested that the IMCI assessment tasks needed improvement. Of those caretakers who had been given or prescribed antimicrobials, 56% knew how to give them to their children correctly when they left the facility, suggesting that the quality of counselling also needed improvement. Almost all (95%) facilities had all essential vaccines available and 62% had all IMCI essential drugs.

The survey did not measure the frequency of supervisory visits, but reports from field staff suggested that supervisory visits to primary health care facilities were not being conducted regularly due to a lack of resources, including vehicles and fuel[11]. Post-training follow up visits were also not always being conducted

[11] Mongolia Short Programme Review, 2007

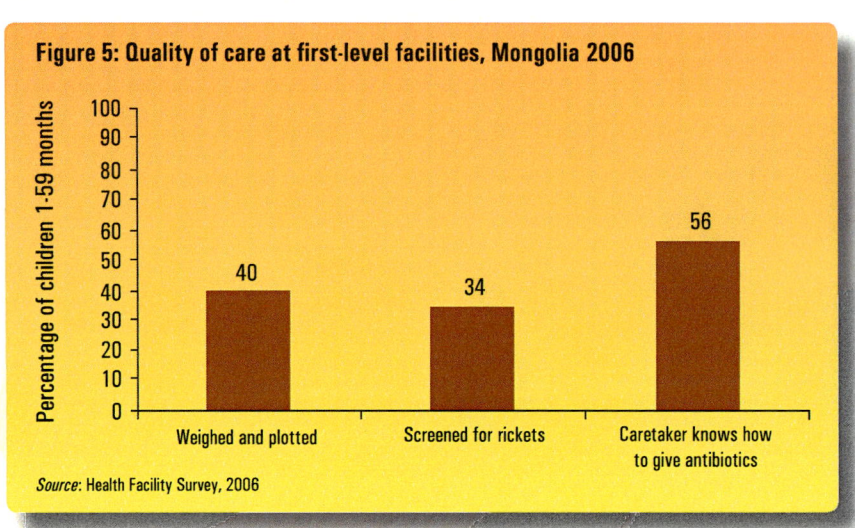

Figure 5: Quality of care at first-level facilities, Mongolia 2006
Source: Health Facility Survey, 2006

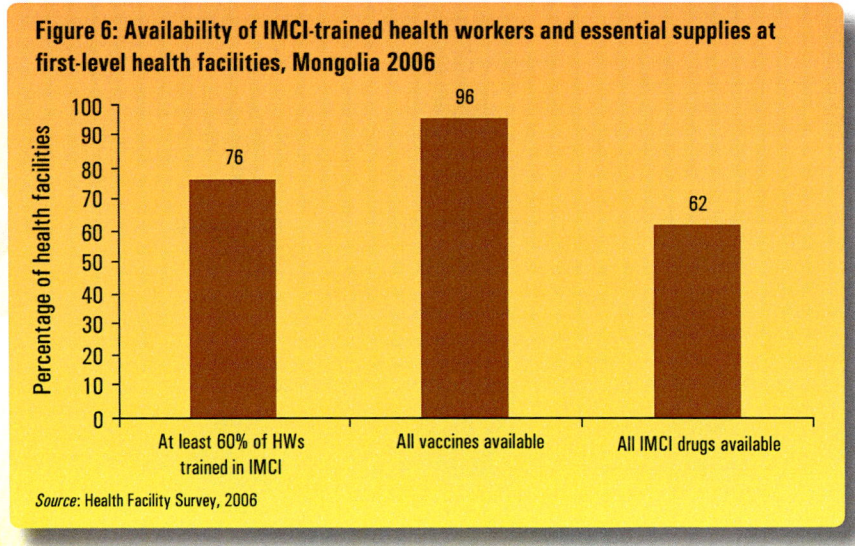

Figure 6: Availability of IMCI-trained health workers and essential supplies at first-level health facilities, Mongolia 2006
Source: Health Facility Survey, 2006

for similar reasons. When supervision was being conducted, it often did not include the use of checklists or observations of clinical practice. Feedback and problem-solving were often not done by supervisors. Staff also reported that essential equipment was sometimes unavailable at peripheral facilities. Equipment that was reported to be often unavailable included oxygen at referral sites, and bags and masks for newborn resuscitation. Referral was generally working well since transportation and services are provided by the Government. However, referral remained more difficult for remote and migratory populations who must travel long distances.

Programme staff also reported that medications were often being sold to the caretakers of children by pharmacists and drug vendors, without prescriptions. The inappropriate use of medications, particularly antibiotics, is believed to be common. Caretakers often seek care from drug sellers before going to government facilities that do not provide drugs free of charge.

The health facility survey and discussions with staff highlighted the following issues as regards quality of care at first-level facilities:

- **Clinical care needed improvement**. Data indicated that not all IMCI assessment tasks were being completed, and that caretakers were not receiving adequate counselling on how to give antibiotics.

- **Supervision needed improvement**. Problems with clinical practice were thought to be related to a lack of regular high quality supervision. Improvements are needed in both the resources available for visits and the skills of supervisors.

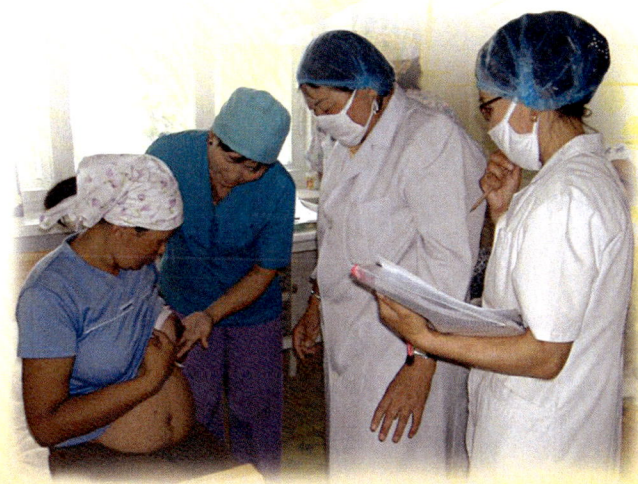

- **Vaccine and drug supply were relatively good in most facilities**. IMCI essential drugs were not available in all facilities, suggesting that health workers need to monitor supplies more actively. Drug management and ordering procedures may need to be reviewed.

- **Referral was working well in most cases**. Remote populations still need more assistance to reach referral sites in a timely fashion.

An evaluation of hospital care was conducted in district, inter-*soum* and *soum* hospitals in 2007. The assessment found that children were often not being triaged efficiently and that health staff were not always aware of up-to-date case-management guidelines. Most hospitals had oxygen available for use by paediatric patients. An emergency triage assessment and treatment course was conducted in 2008 for a core set of trainers, and the child health guidelines in the WHO *Pocket book of hospital care for children* were adapted.

Lessons learnt: Health systems

Emphasize access to and quality of IMCI services

- Access to health services is high for many essential services. Poor, rural and migratory populations have less access and need to be better reached. Problems relating to staff availability and the financing of drugs at first-level facilities should be addressed by policy-makers.

- Health facility surveys are useful for reviewing the quality of clinical care and the facility supports required to improve care at first-level facilities.

- The clinical skills of health workers need to be reinforced continuously after training. Both the number and quality of supervisory visits to peripheral areas need to be improved.

- Inappropriate prescribing of medications by pharmacists and drug-sellers is a problem in many areas.

6.4 Improving the coverage of child health interventions

The primary objective of IMCI is to improve population coverage with effective child health interventions. Child health interventions are treatments, technologies and key health behaviours that prevent or treat child illness and reduce deaths in children under five years of age. Interventions that are included in the child health programme in Mongolia are summarized in the box on the next page.

Interventions are usually delivered using a combination of: (1) services (to provide preventive and treatment interventions); (2) health education (to improve knowledge and behaviours); (3) distribution of essential commodities (iodized salt); and (4) infrastructure (such as transportation for referral).

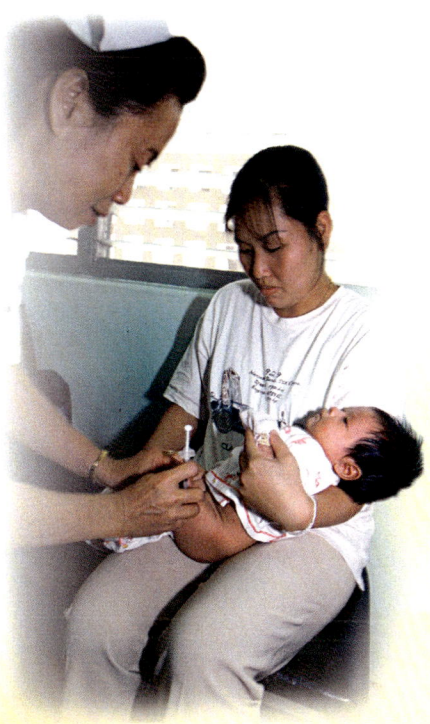

Many of these interventions are included as a part of IMCI at the facility and community level. Vaccines are delivered by the Expanded Programme on Immunization (EPI) programme. Maternal and early newborn interventions are part of the maternal health programme and are delivered through antenatal, delivery and immediate post-delivery contacts.

Interventions that are currently implemented by the child health programme in Mongolia

Newborn period (1 hour after birth – 28 days)

Preventive
- Early initiation of breastfeeding and exclusive breastfeeding
- Thermal care
- Hygienic cord care

Treatment
- Prompt care-seeking for illness
- Management of diarrhoea, feeding problems and low weight
- Identification of severe illness
- Emergency management of severe newborn illness—infections, asphyxia, preterm birth

Childhood (1-59 months)

Preventive
- Exclusive breastfeeding (6 months), continued breastfeeding (6-24 months)
- Safe and appropriate complementary feeding
- EPI vaccines (BCG, hepatitis B, DPT, OPV, measles)
- Vitamin A
- Iodine
- Vitamin D

Treatment
- Oral rehydration therapy for diarrhoea
- Antibiotics for dysentery
- Antibiotics for pneumonia

Strategy/programmes used to deliver interventions

IMCI – facility-based
IMCI – community-based (promotion of key newborn and child health behaviours)
EPI
Nutrition
Maternal and newborn health

Coverage with newborn interventions

In the area of newborn care, the IMCI approach emphasizes exclusive breastfeeding, early recognition of and care-seeking for newborn illness, and management of sick newborns. No data are available on referral or case-management practices for sick newborns. Newborn sepsis remains a relatively small component of newborn deaths, with the highest proportion attributed to asphyxia and prematurity.

- **Breastfeeding in the first hour after delivery**. In 2008, 81% of women reported that they breastfed their neonate in the first hour after delivery[12]—a key nutritional intervention—suggesting that the importance of such behaviour is being emphasized (see Figure 7). A high proportion of births in Mongolia are attended by skilled birth attendants (99% in 2008)[13], who also usually provide care in the immediate newborn period, supported through the maternal programme. The presence of skilled providers at delivery is an important step towards improving the quality of care in the immediate newborn period. No data are yet available on how well other interventions in this period are delivered. Immediate newborn care interventions include appropriate thermal care and cord-cutting, as well as management of life-threatening conditions at delivery, such as asphyxia and prematurity. The high proportion of newborn deaths attributed to asphyxia and prematurity suggests that the quality of both antenatal and delivery care needs improvement.

- **Follow-up visit in the first seven days of life**. In 2008, 65% of mothers received a follow-up visit in the first seven days—a rate that is much lower than the proportion of deliveries attended by a skilled provider. The early follow-up rate

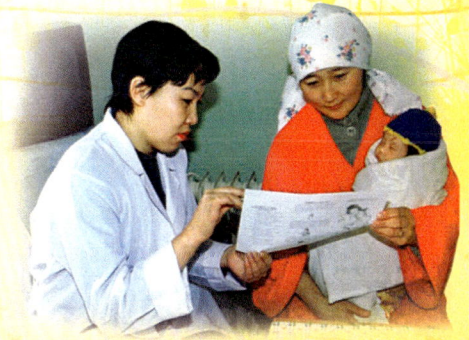

[12] UNFPA RHS, 2008
[13] Ibid

needs to be improved. The risk of newborn death is highest in the early newborn period, with the majority of deaths happening in the first seven days of life. For this reason, care contacts in the early newborn period are emphasized. Such contacts allow babies to be screened for feeding problems and for signs of illness, and referred or managed if necessary. They also allow health education messages on newborn care to be given. Since most births are attended by skilled providers in Mongolia, most babies receive care contacts immediately after delivery, and in the first 24 hours. At least one follow-up visit in the first seven days of life is then recommended.

- **Exclusive breastfeeding in the first month of life**. Ninety-five percent of newborns in Mongolia are being exclusively breastfed in the first month of life, which is a very high coverage rate (see Figure 7). Exclusive breastfeeding during this period is important for both nutrition and the prevention of infections. High rates of exclusive breastfeeding during this period suggest that this practice is being reinforced by delivery staff and by health education.

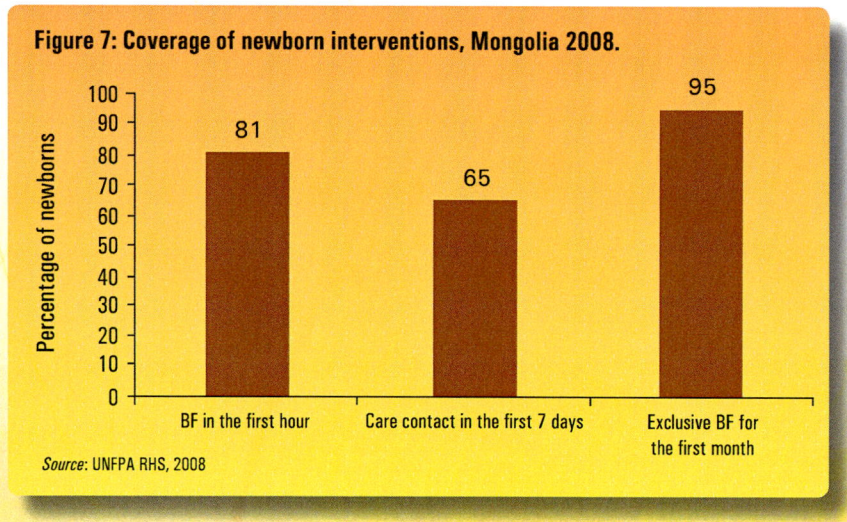

Figure 7: Coverage of newborn interventions, Mongolia 2008.

Source: UNFPA RHS, 2008

Coverage with child interventions

- **Exclusive breastfeeding.** The prevalence of exclusive breastfeeding drops for older infants, with the rate estimated to be 79% of infants up to six months of age in 2008[14] (see Figure 8). Twenty-one per cent of women do not exclusively breastfeed for the full recommended period. There are a number of possible reasons for this, including time constraints (the need to look after other children and to work) and the use of breast-milk substitutes. More information is needed on the barriers to exclusive breastfeeding for the full six months. The duration in the definition of exclusive breastfeeding was changed in Mongolia in 2002, from four to six months.

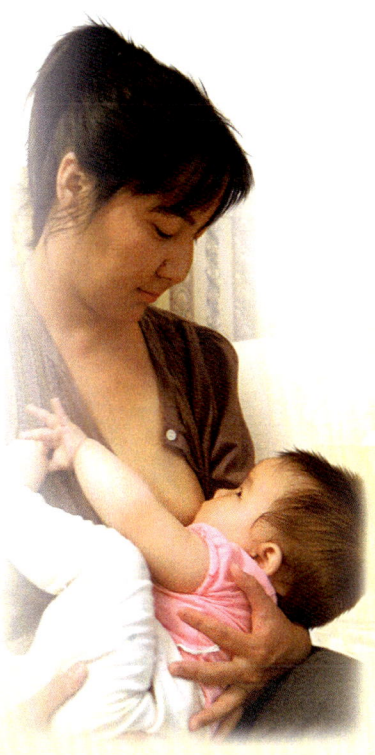

- **Complementary feeding.** The proportion of infants aged six to nine months who receive appropriate breastfeeding and complementary feeding was estimated to be 82% in 2008[15] (see Figure 8). This indicator is defined as the proportion of infants aged six to nine months who receive breast milk and solid or semi-solid foods, and is based on a 24-hour dietary recall. The high rates of stunting suggest that feeding practices around the time of weaning need to be improved. In order to improve complementary feeding practices, data are needed on three important elements of

[14] UNFPA RHS, 2008
[15] *Ibid*

feeding: (1) the quality of the food that is being offered to children (energy density, micronutrient composition, food handling); (2) the quantity of food given; and (3) the frequency of feeding. The recommended frequency for infants aged six to eight months is twice daily and three times daily for those aged nine to 11 months. More data are needed in order to develop better counselling messages or other methods for improving practice.

- **Vitamin A**. The proportion of children who had received a dose of vitamin A in the previous six months was 65% in 2005[16], and has shown an upward trend since 2000, when the reported coverage was 32%. This suggests that the distribution of vitamin A capsules is improving. More effort is still required.

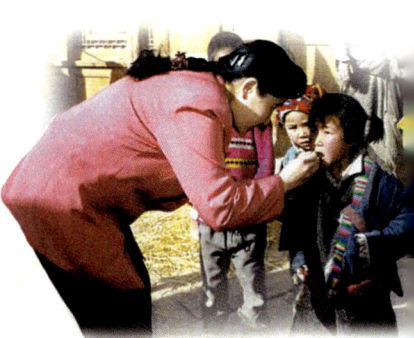

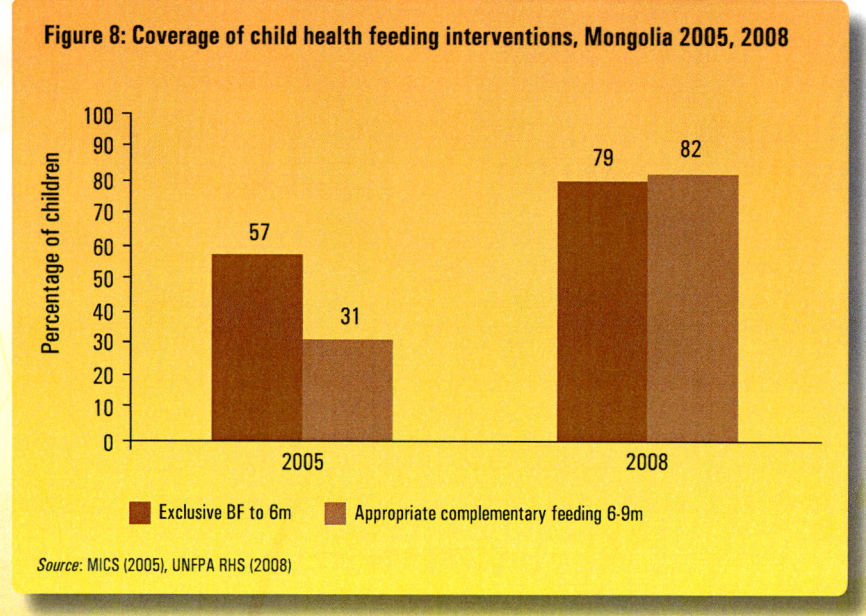

Figure 8: Coverage of child health feeding interventions, Mongolia 2005, 2008

Source: MICS (2005), UNFPA RHS (2008)

[16]MICS, 2005

- **Use of iodized salt**. The proportion of households using iodized salt was estimated to be 74% in 2004, an upward trend from 1999, when coverage was estimated to be 44%[17]. Western regions of the country had lower coverage than all other areas. Overall, the use of iodized salt has shown significant improvement.

- **Vitamin D**. In 2004, it was estimated that 16% of children under two years of age had received 50 000 IU of vitamin D in the previous 12 months. Vitamin D coverage needs improvement.

- **Fully vaccinated children**. The proportion of children fully vaccinated by 12 months of age against measles, DPT, polio and hepatitis B was estimated to be 98% in 2006 from routine data, but only 67% from the 2005 UNICEF Multiple Indicator Cluster Survey. Coverage is high for vaccines that are given early in life, such as BCG, DPT and polio. Measles vaccine tends to be given late, with 76% of children receiving measles before 12 months of age, and 15% receiving it after 12 months.[18] Regional variations in vaccination coverage are noted, with western areas of the country tending to have lower coverage rates.

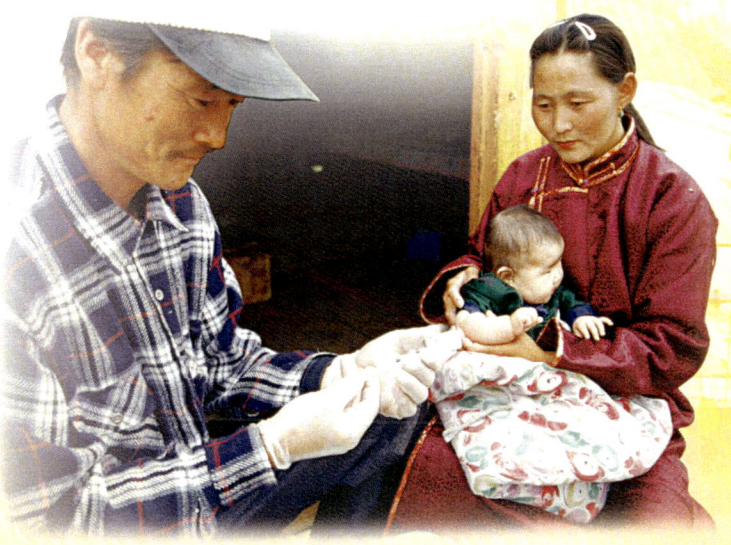

[17]National NS, 1999 and 2004
[18]MICS, 2005

- **Oral Rehydration Therapy (ORT) for diarrhoea.** The proportion of children receiving ORT for diarrhoea was 83% in 2008[19]. ORT use rate was estimated to be 63% in the 2005 MICS. It is encouraging that the use of oral fluids for the management of diarrhoea has improved. ORT includes ORS and/or recommended home fluids (RHF), and is the most cost-effective approach for prevention of dehydration (see Figure 9).

- **Treatment of pneumonia.** 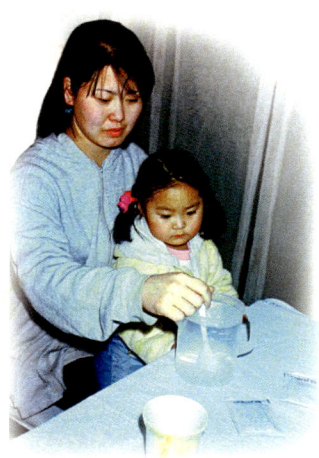 The proportion of children with suspected pneumonia taken to an appropriate provider for treatment was 63% in 2005, an increase from the 47% calculated by the 2000 MICS. In 2005, 71% of children with suspected pneumonia received antibiotics. Going to an appropriate provider for treatment is assumed to be a proxy measure of quality of care. Children taken to trained providers

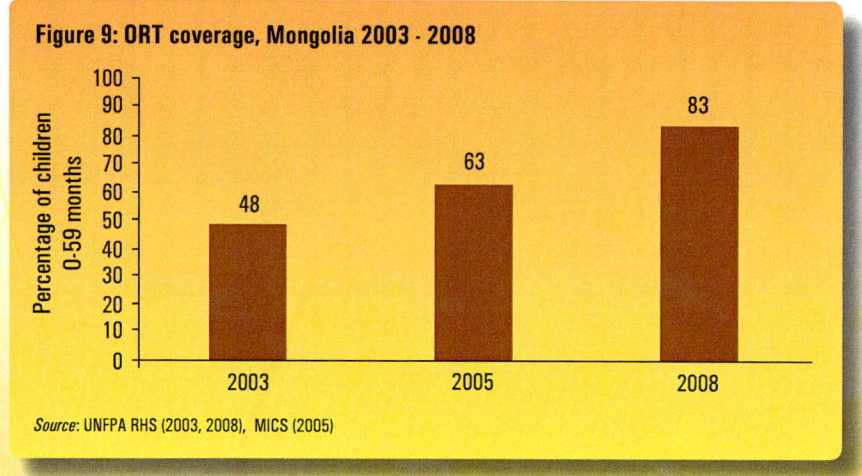

Figure 9: ORT coverage, Mongolia 2003 - 2008

Source: UNFPA RHS (2003, 2008), MICS (2005)

[19] UNFPA RHS, 2008

are more likely to be appropriately assessed and classified, and those needing antibiotics are more likely to receive an appropriate antibiotic.

- **Support therapy for sick children**. The proportion of sick children offered increased fluids and continued feeding was 72% in 2008, as compared to previous estimates in 1998 (62%) and 2003 (76%)[20]. Increased fluids and continued feeding are considered support measures for sick children to prevent dehydration and weight loss.

- **Care-seeking practice**. The proportion of caretakers knowing at least two danger signs for seeking care immediately for a child with suspected pneumonia was 81% in the 2005 MICS. In that survey, questions regarding knowledge of general danger signs for sick children were not asked, but the survey found that 86% of mothers and caretakers would seek immediate care for a child with fever, but only 21% would do so for a child with fast breathing and 23% for a child with difficulty in breathing (see Figure 10). Knowledge of danger signs is important for encouraging early care-seeking for sick children.

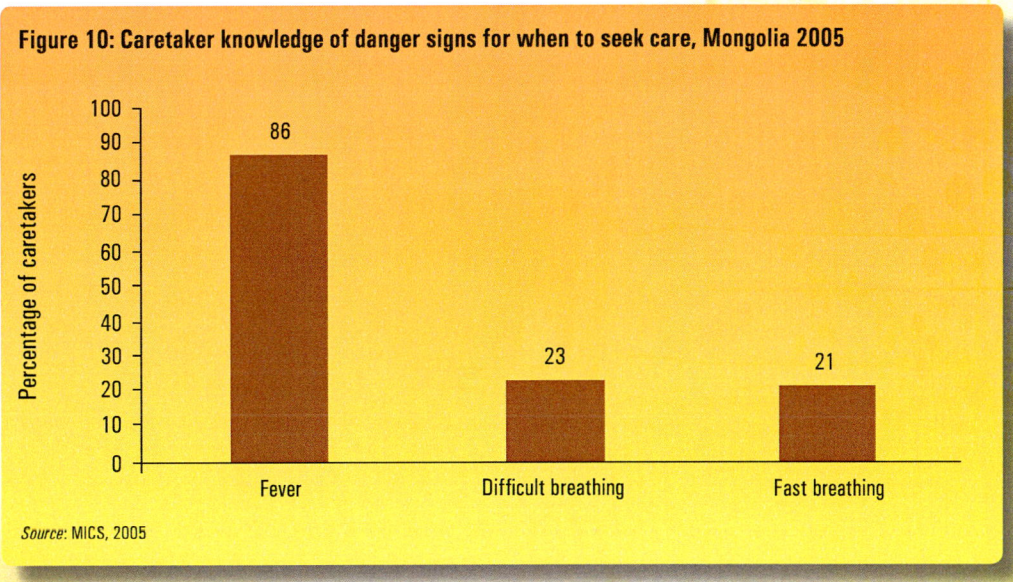

Figure 10: Caretaker knowledge of danger signs for when to seek care, Mongolia 2005

Source: MICS, 2005

[20] UNFPA Reproductive Health Survey 1998, 2003, 2008

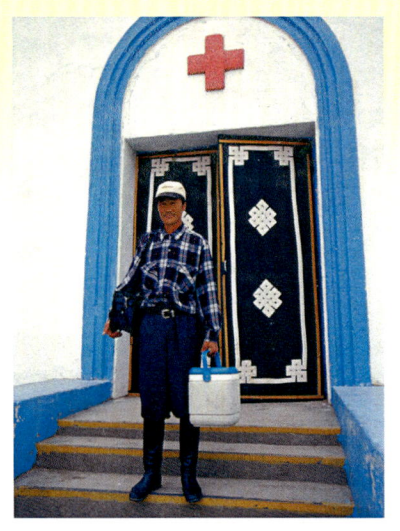

"We have found that the practices of mothers in the villages have not improved as quickly as we expected. Feldshers go out to the villages. In most areas they reach households. But they may not be doing enough to change what mothers do. We can see that more needs to be done to change the health practices of mothers and their families." Soum nurse

Approaches for improving intervention coverage

Three main approaches have been used to improve the child health knowledge and practices of families and communities:

- **Household visits by *bagh feldshers***. Each f*eldsher* is responsible for approximately 300 households. *Feldshers* provide regular, door-to-door visits and deliver health education and primary health care services. They use the mother's card for health education, and may have other additional counselling materials. Historically, the *feldsher* system has been highly organized and effective in reaching all communities. Household visits and direct one-on-one counselling have been seen as the most effective communication approach.

- **Health facility contacts**. Health workers provide health education whenever caretakers bring their children for preventive care or treatment. Materials used include the IMCI mother's card, and health education posters.

- **Mass and print media**. The National Center for Health Development is the main national organization responsible for health promotion and communication. They have developed information, education and communication materials, including materials for airing on television and radio spots. IMCI messages and materials for parents and health workers have also been developed. Most health education material development has been funded by donors. Government resources are not routinely available for mass and print media.

Coverage data show that key health behaviours have improved in the last five years. Feeding practices, however, particularly complementary feeding, need further improvement. Discussions with staff at all levels[21] highlighted areas where more attention is needed, including:

- **Improving the availability of trained *feldshers***. As discussed in the training section, 90 *baghs* had no *feldsher* available in 2006. More *feldshers* are needed.

- **Improving the quality and availability of health education materials**. Health education materials need improvement, particularly in the area of nutrition. Messages should focus on improving key child health behaviours. They should use language that is understandable to people in different areas of the country. Materials should be easy to use and should use pictures that help to convey messages. All messages and materials should be field-tested. Health staff should have education materials available for use. In order to decide how messages can be improved, more data are needed in order to understand perceptions about particular behaviours, and the barriers to changing them.

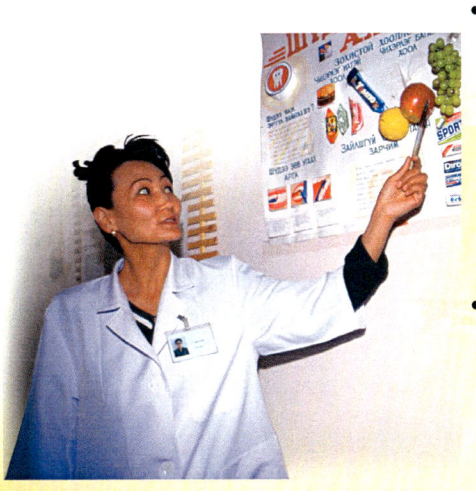

- **Improving the counselling skills of health workers**. Health workers often have little training and experience in the area of counselling. More training and supervision in this area would be useful.

- **Reviewing the channels and methods used for health education**. Wider use of mass or print media may be useful in reaching some communities more

[21]Mongolia Short Programme Review, 2007

effectively. Alternative methods of conducting nutrition education in communities, such as peer-to-peer methods, could be used more widely.

- **Reviewing community involvement with child health activities**. Available resources in communities are not always being used to educate and reinforce important child health behaviours. Community resources that could be better used include NGOs, teachers and community leaders. A strategy for linking community resources with child health is needed.

Lessons learnt: Improving intervention coverage

Emphasize improved knowledge and practices of caretakers and families

- Good progress has been made in improving the coverage of child health interventions in several areas, including breastfeeding initiation, vaccinations, distribution of iodine and vitamin A, care-seeking for pneumonia and treatment of diarrhoea.

- More work is needed to improve exclusive breastfeeding and complementary feeding practices and knowledge of danger signs.

- The methods and materials used for health education need to be reviewed regularly. The review should include the effectiveness of the health education messages and the availability of education materials, as well as the most effective methods for reaching caretakers and families.
  More research is needed on barriers to changing some types of behaviour, particularly feeding.

- Approaches to improving the counselling skills of IMCI-trained health workers are needed.

- New strategies for reaching communities should be developed. These could include ensuring that enough trained *feldshers* are available and improving the involvement of community leaders and groups in child health activities.

6.5 Monitoring and evaluating progress

A number of methods have been used to monitor and evaluate the IMCI strategy in Mongolia. Effective monitoring and evaluation has been important in making planning decisions. The methods that have been used are summarized below.

Household surveys

Household surveys have been used to evaluate the knowledge and practices of caretakers as regards the prevention and treatment of illness in children and newborn babies and to assess the coverage of child health interventions. Three types of survey have been conducted in Mongolia: the UNICEF Multiple Indicator Cluster Survey, the United Nations Population Fund Reproductive Health Survey, and the National Nutrition Survey. These surveys calculate standard child health indicators, and all use a national sampling frame. Data collected can be disaggregated to the *aimag* level so that different regions can be compared. Surveys have been conducted every three to five years and have been essential for reviewing progress at the population level.

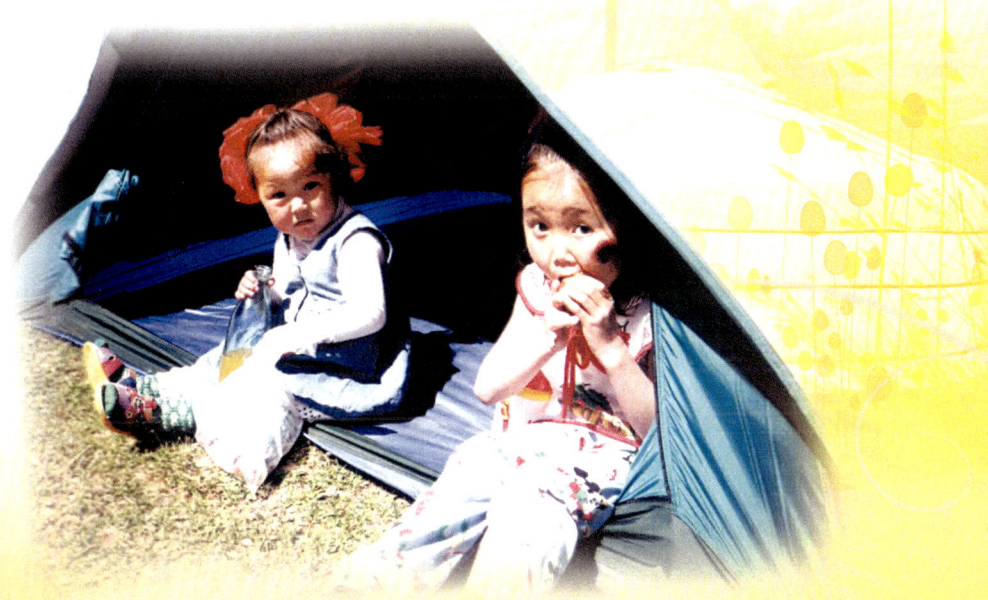

Experience with household surveys has shown the following:

- Additional data are needed in some areas, including newborn practices, distribution of iron to children, treatment of ARI with antibiotics, and inappropriate prescribing of antibiotics and other medications by the private sector. Questions on these issues need to be added to future surveys. Definitions should be consistent with those used internationally and recommended in the WHO/UNICEF Regional Child Survival Strategy.

- Household data are not always useful for low-level planning because they cannot be disaggregated to levels below the *aimag*. In order to collect local data, smaller sample, 30-cluster household surveys could be used.

- *Aimag* planners still need more experience with the interpretation and use of population-based data for planning activities. Reaching families and communities has proved to be the most challenging part of implementation.

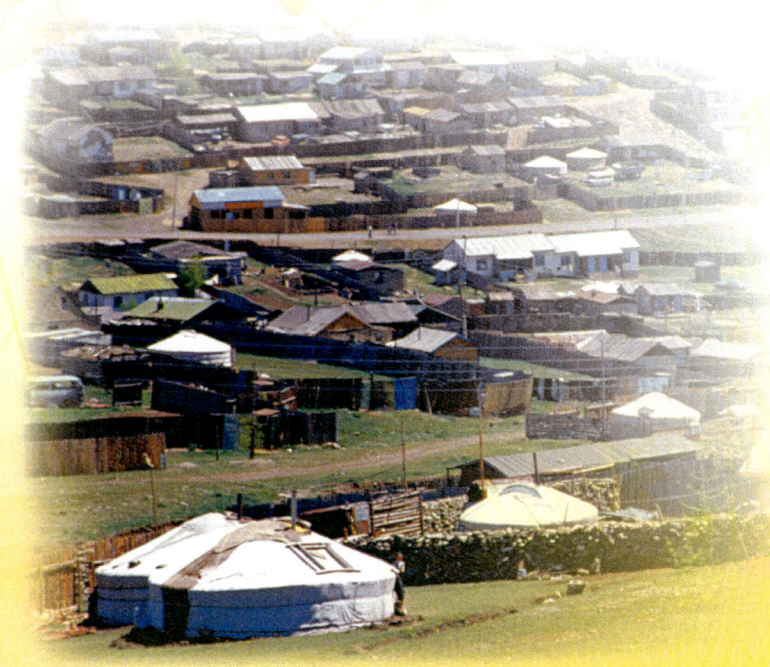

Health facility surveys

Health facility surveys have been used to evaluate the quality of care provided at first and referral-level health facilities that have implemented IMCI. Facility surveys provide the best quality field data on case-management practices and the availability of facility support. A standard protocol, including standard checklists, is used. The surveys observe elements of case-management practice for sick children, as well as reviewing drugs, equipment and supplies. Interviews with caretakers and health workers are also often included. A team of surveyors is trained in the survey methods. Data are summarized as key facility-based indicators and then discussed and interpreted by local staff. These data are useful for identifying gaps and planning activities for improving training and follow-up. WHO has developed an IMCI health facility tool that has been tested and used in a number of different countries, as well as a tool for measuring the quality of hospital care.

Experience with health facility surveys has shown:

- Facility surveys should always include validation of the health worker's assessment and classification of illness by a trained IMCI observer, to allow observers to decide whether or not health workers have treated cases correctly.
- Improvements in the quality of care require improved follow-up after training and improved supervisory practices. It is difficult to sustain improvements in practice without regular review and support of health workers. In the longer term, it is hoped that the quality of IMCI will be improved by pre-service training of health staff.

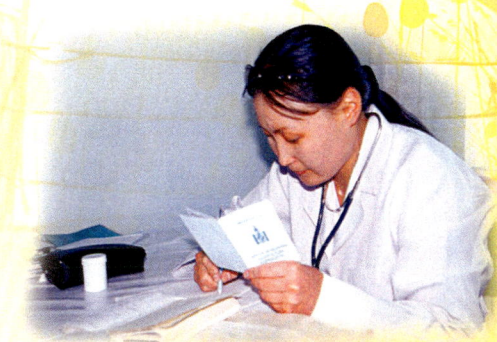

- Facility surveys should be done regularly. Only one IMCI survey and one hospital assessment have been conducted since the expansion phase of IMCI began in Mongolia. Ideally, surveys should be conducted every two to three years, to provide regular data for planning.

Routine reporting system

The routine reporting system is used to collect data regularly from all or most facilities in the country. Data are collected in a number of areas including: births and deaths (vital registration), cases seen, treatment received and vaccinations given. Rates are calculated using data on the total number of children, taken from civil records. Civil registration law in Mongolia requires that a child be registered within 15 days of birth in urban areas and 30 days in rural areas. Birth registration is free of charge. The 2005 MICS found that 98% of children under five were registered. Eighty-six per cent of mothers were able to show a birth certificate while 13%, although unable to show the certificate, reported that they had one. There were no significant variations in birth registration by sex, region and education. Overall, birth registration is believed to be relatively complete. No data are available on the completeness of death registration. Routine data report only on cases coming to health facilities. It is recognized that facility-based data will miss cases or deaths that occur outside health facilities. In addition, the calculation of rates from facility-based data requires that denominators—estimates of the number of infants and children—are accurate.

Experience with routine data has shown:

- Routine data are useful for local planning, since they are available for the *soum* level and are collected continuously.

- No data are available on the quality of routine data. There are a number of factors that could decrease the validity and reliability of data, including the completeness of record-keeping, how cases are classified, and the accuracy of denominators. Estimates of local populations using community birth and death records may not be accurate, particularly in areas where there is a large migratory population. Routine data are most useful for following trends over time, rather than making statements about absolute rates.

- The routine system does not yet record cases using IMCI case definitions. Use of these definitions would make record-keeping easier at the facility level, and would reinforce the use of IMCI case-management. In addition, IMCI-trained health workers may be more likely to mis-classify cases if they have to record cases using different classifications.

Annual review and planning meetings with *aimag* staff

As mentioned in the planning section, regular planning with local staff provides a good opportunity to review available data, progress with workplans, problems and gaps. This has proved to be a useful method for monitoring progress over time. Routine Health Management Information System data are used, as well as reports on activities conducted.

Short programme review for child health

A short programme review (SPR) was conducted in May 2007. An SPR is a method of systematically reviewing all aspects of child health programming and determining how well activities have been implemented. Main problems are identified, and recommendations for the next workplan are developed.

In Mongolia, the SPR was conducted in five days. It was designed to build on the existing process of routine programme planning and reviewed child health-related activities at the pregnancy and delivery periods, as well as those directed at newborn babies, infants and older children (the continuum of care for the mother and child). This broader scope was felt to be important, in order to maximize the programme's impact on overall child survival.

The SPR was conducted by the Ministry of Health in collaboration with WHO. It was attended by Ministry staff from the central, provincial and *soum* levels, staff from the Public Health Institute, the University of Medical Sciences and the Nutrition Research Centre, and staff from partner organizations involved in child health programming—ADB, the Norwegian Lutheran Mission, UNICEF, UNFPA, WHO and World Vision. The Ministry of Health staff included representatives from child health, nutrition, reproductive health and the expanded programme on immunization.

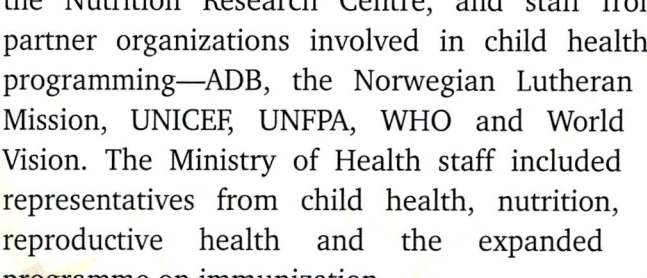

The SPR process proved to be useful because it:

- brought staff from different levels together (input from those working on the ground was particularly useful for understanding what was really happening in the field);
- brought staff from different programme areas together (a number of different programmes are responsible for child health activities – joint planning meant that activities were better coordinated);
- involved stakeholders (local partners were able to explain what they had observed and what they were doing. All stakeholders were able to see where more work was needed. Resource needs were discussed); and
- led to concrete recommendations for action that could be implemented in the next workplan.

In the longer term, it is hoped that this type of review can be done regularly.

Lessons learnt: Monitoring and evaluation

Apply appropriate methods and use data to make programme decisions

- Household surveys are essential for collecting population-based data on intervention coverage. Care should be taken that surveys collect data on standard indicators.
- Facility surveys are essential for collecting data on the quality of care at health facilities. Surveys should include re-examination of children by a trained observer to determine whether or not health workers have classified and treated children correctly.
- Routine data are useful for ongoing monitoring. The quality of the data collected will vary depending on a number of factors, including the accuracy of denominators. Routine data are useful for tracking trends over time.
- Regular planning with *aimag* staff allows data to be reviewed and local staff to give input on progress at low levels—both quantitative and qualitative information is used.
- The SPR method is useful for evaluating progress periodically and making recommendations for the future with staff from different programmes and stakeholders. Data and field experience are taken into account.

7 Directions for the Future

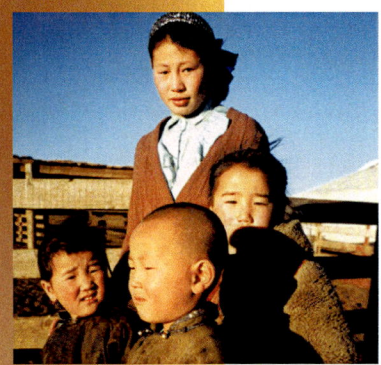

"We feel that IMCI has been successfully introduced in Mongolia. We have achieved a great deal and learnt a great deal. The key has been strong collaboration between our partners and health workers at all levels of the health system. More remains to be done, but we feel that we have the skills to make improvements. A particular focus will be working on improving knowledge and practices in the community."
IMCI focal person, Ulaanbaatar

IMCI has been successfully implemented in Mongolia. Training coverage is high and there have been positive outcomes in a number of areas, including measures of quality of care and coverage with child health interventions. A system for monitoring and evaluating progress has been put in place. Planning is being done collaboratively with field staff and stakeholders. Future efforts will continue to improve the quality of implementation in several key areas.

Quality of behaviour change and communication

Improving the knowledge and practices of caretakers in key areas will continue to be a focus of IMCI—including exclusive breastfeeding, complementary feeding, consumption of adequate micronutrients and home care for sick children. Although counselling materials are generally available, the quality of counselling and health education could be improved. The approach to behaviour change will be reviewed, including the technical quality of the materials and messages used, the channels used to deliver messages, and how to strengthen counselling practices. New messages on the use of drugs sold by private drug vendors may be needed. More research is needed to understand some types of behaviour, and the barriers to changing them.

Community

The good community-based system using *feldshers* to visit households and provide education and referral is widespread. There are concerns, however, that inadequate numbers of *feldshers* are being trained—some communities no longer have active *feldshers* available. Improved community mobilization is needed in order to ensure transportation for women and children needing referral. Improved community awareness of key health behaviours may also encourage support for appropriate health practices in the home and community. Greater advocacy for improved community involvement is needed. *Feldsher* training and posting needs to be reviewed at a high level.

Access to care

Although access to care is high for most of the population, it is still limited for some groups, including some rural and migratory populations. More advocacy aimed at policy-makers is needed to highlight that problem and to seek policies to address the training and retention of health staff, as well as the barriers to registering for health care or paying for medicines.

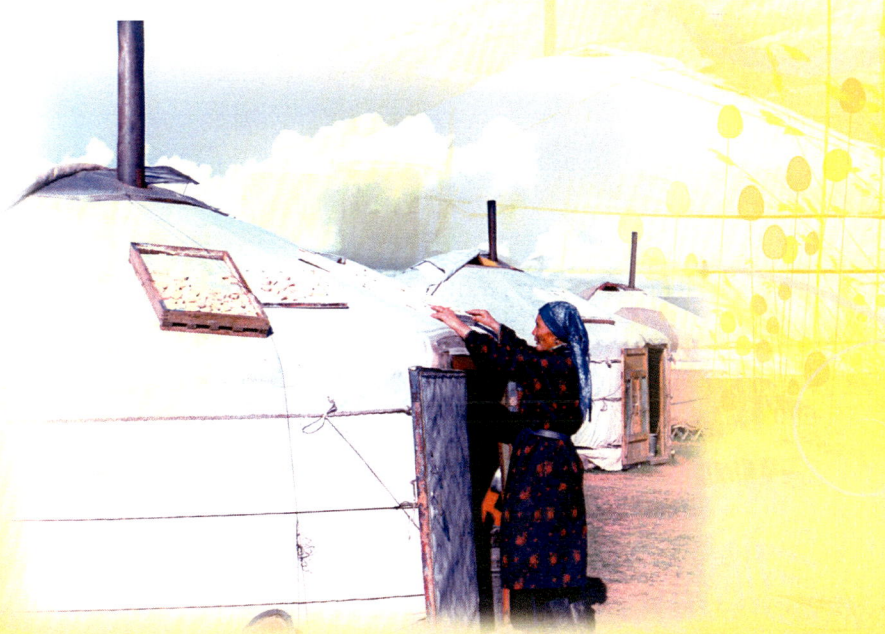

Quality of care

Follow-up after training and supervision of health workers needs to be strengthened. National and *aimag* staff need to investigate strategies to make this happen. Donors may be able to contribute financial and technical resources. A follow-up health facility survey is needed to assess progress. Methods of evaluating the quality of IMCI follow-up after training are needed.

Availability and use of data

More data are needed in some key areas, including the quality of newborn care, the management of severely ill newborn babies and children, the distribution of iron to children, the treatment of ARI, and the role of private prescribers in the treatment of children. Such data would be useful for programme planning and future household surveys will include indicators in these areas. An approach to improving the use of data for planning by *aimag* managers is also needed.

Lessons learnt: Directions for the future

- Improving the knowledge and behaviour of caretakers needs further emphasis, including review of the messages and materials used and the methods used to transmit messages.
- Improving community involvement in promoting child health needs continued emphasis.
- Access to care for some groups in the population needs to be emphasized in advocacy messages, and policies to improve access need to be revised and improved.
- Improving the quality of care through regular follow-up and supervision will receive continued attention.
- Data from household and facility surveys will continue to play an important role in making programme decisions. Data collected by surveys will be updated and revised to ensure that all key indicators are measured.
- Use of data for local planning will be strengthened.

Acknowledgement

The main contributors to this document were: John Murray, consultant and principal author; Gochoo Soyolgerel, Ministry of Health, Mongolia; Emmalita Mañalac and Marianna Trias, Maternal, Child Health and Nutrition of the World Health Organization Regional Office for the Western Pacific.

The team gratefully acknowledges the technical review made by Patria Angos, Naor Bar-Zeev and Angelica Flores-Verschoor and the secretarial assistance of Liza Clavecilla. Roslyn Stirling edited the document. Design and layout were done by EC2C Media Production.